Table of Contents

URTICARIA

Maintaining Clear Skin: A Comprehensive Strategy for Urticaria Wellness

CHAD BRUNO

Introductory

Urticarial, more popularly known as hives, is a skin disorder characterized by the abrupt onset of wheals or welts that are red, elevated, and irritating. The size and appearance of these welts can change rapidly, sometimes within just a few hours. Chronic urticaria lasts more than six weeks, while acute urticaria lasts anywhere from a few hours to six weeks. An allergic reaction to something like food, medication, insect stings, or environmental variables is usually what sets it off. Urticaria can also occur for no apparent reason in certain people. The disorder is the result of histamine and other chemicals being released in the skin, causing to the distinctive itching and welts. Medication, such as antihistamines, may be used to treat symptoms and get to the bottom of what's causing them.

CHAPTER ONE
Urticaria's Repercussions

The consequences of urticaria, often known as hives, depend on the condition's intensity, how long it lasts, and the patient's general health. Urticaria can have a wide range of effects on sufferers, including:

• Urticaria causes itching, burning, and stinging sensations, all of which are physically unpleasant. Pain is a possible side effect in severe cases.

• Hives, or urticaria, are characterized by red, raised welts that can be unpleasant and have an impact on a person's self-esteem and body image, especially if they are chronic or recurrent.

• Irritation and exhaustion are common results of a lack of sleep caused by hives.

• The emotional toll of dealing with persistent symptoms of chronic urticaria, as well as the condition's unpredictable character, can lead to stress, anxiety, and depression.

• Urticaria can have a negative effect on a person's day-to-day life, including their ability to work and exercise, depending on the degree and location of the hives.

• In terms of one's social life, urticaria's outwardly apparent symptoms may cause one to withdraw from activities for fear of ridicule or pain.

• Costs connected with treatment for chronic urticaria, such as medical appointments, medications, and possible changes to one's way of life, might be prohibitive.

• **Secondary infections:** Scratching hives can damage the skin, increasing the risk of infections.

Acute urticaria typically goes away on its own, and its effects can be lessened with the right therapy.

Effective management of chronic urticaria requires first determining and then fixing the underlying causes. Individuals can lessen the effects of urticaria and boost their quality of life by working together with a healthcare physician, allergist, or dermatologist to design a treatment plan.

Chronic Itchy Rash

Hives, or urticaria, can be broken down into different subtypes based on parameters such as severity, triggers, and clinical presentation. Urticaria comes in a variety of forms, including:

1. Acute urticaria is characterized by a relatively brief duration, usually under six weeks. Common triggers include allergens in food or medication, as well as stings from insects. In most cases, antihistamines and other therapies are all that's needed to get rid of acute urticaria.

2. Urticaria that lasts longer than six weeks is considered chronic and may continue for months or even years. It's more difficult to pin down a definitive reason, which could be autoimmune, physical, or some other underlying component.

The symptoms of chronic urticaria can make daily activities difficult.

3. Physical Urticaria: This type of urticaria is produced by physical stimuli or conditions, such as pressure on the skin, cold or heat exposure, sun exposure (solar urticaria), vibration (vibratory urticaria), or friction (dermographism). The welts appear near the source of the physical provocation and may not last long.

4. Skin gets raised and red when scratched or lightly stroked; this condition is known as dermatographism and is a form of physical urticaria. It's a type of physical urticaria that shows up frequently.

5. An increase in core body temperature, as may occur during perspiration, physical exertion, or emotional stress, is the inciting factor in cholinergic urticaria. It causes severe itching and pinpoint hives.

6. For those who suffer with aquagenic urticaria, any contact with water, no matter how cold or hot, will result in an outbreak of hives. This is a rare condition.

7. An allergy to cold temperatures causes cold urticaria. Hives are caused by a reduction in body temperature, no matter how minor, and can be fatal in extreme circumstances.

8. Some people who suffer from chronic urticaria have an autoimmune reaction in which their immune system mistakenly assaults healthy tissues in the body. Autoantibodies that attack mast cells in the skin have been linked to autoimmune urticaria.

9. Idiopathic Urticaria: When the etiology of urticaria cannot be determined, it is referred to as idiopathic urticaria. This occurs frequently in cases of chronic urticaria where no obvious cause can be pinpointed.

Because the diagnosis and treatment of urticaria might vary according to the exact kind and underlying causes, it is crucial to seek medical examination and guidance. Urticaria sufferers should consult a doctor, allergist, or dermatologist for advice on the best course of treatment.

Hives, or urticaria, can have several potential causes or triggers. Understanding the underlying reason or trigger is key for properly managing and treating the illness. **The following are examples of common causes and triggers of urticaria**:

• Common triggers for urticaria include allergens and chemical or food sensitivities. Foods (such as nuts, shellfish, eggs), drugs (such as antibiotics and aspirin), insect stings, and environmental allergens (such as pollen and dust mites) can all trigger an allergic reaction in some people.

• Urticaria can be triggered by bacterial or viral infections. For example, the Epstein-Barr virus or hepatitis may be related with urticaria.

• Causes of physical urticaria include, but are not limited to, the following physical stressors or factors:

Scratching or stroking the skin (dermographism).

Urticaria caused by exposure to cold weather.

Urticaria brought on by heat or perspiration.

Urticaria brought on by pressing on the skin (o Pressure Urticaria).

Urticaria from Exposure to Vibrations, or "VU" for short.

• Extreme stress or emotional tension can bring on or exacerbate urticaria in certain people.

• Histamine release and hives are triggered when mast cells are mistakenly attacked by the immune system during an autoimmune reaction, which is linked to some cases of urticaria.

• Many cases of urticaria have idiopathic causes since doctors are unable to pin down a single trigger for the condition.

- Some people have an allergic reaction to food additives such artificial colors and preservatives, which can lead to an outbreak of hives.

- Hives are a common adverse effect to several drugs. Antibiotics, NSAIDs, and other pain medicines are particularly prone to this side effect.

- **Insect Bites and Stings:** Hives can develop at the site of insect bites or stings, especially in persons who are allergic to the venom.

- Urticaria at the site of touch can be caused by an allergic reaction to a contact allergen, such as a plant or chemical.

• Cholinergic urticaria has been linked to physical activity and higher core body temperatures in some people.

• Solar urticaria is an extremely unusual disorder in which hives appear after being exposed to sunshine.

In cases with chronic urticaria, it is crucial to collaborate with a healthcare expert to identify the precise reason or trigger of the condition. Depending on the root reason and the specifics of each case, treatment and management options will be different. Antihistamines and other drugs are often used to treat the symptoms of urticaria and keep the condition under control.

CHAPTER TWO
Most Typical Signs

Wheals or welts of raised, red, itchy skin are the most recognizable sign of urticaria (hives). These welts can vary in size and shape and often come and go over a short period. Common symptoms of urticaria, aside from the welts themselves, include the following:

1. Urticaria is characterized by an intense itching. Itching from the welts and hives is a common symptom and can be very bothersome.

2. Rash: The affected area of skin turns red and swollen.

3. Puffiness may occur because the welts are elevated and create localized swelling.

4. Hives can range in size and shape from small, isolated welts to big, elevated skin patches. Shapes range from spherical to oval to irregular.

5. Hives typically arise within minutes or hours of being exposed to whatever allergen or trigger is causing them.

6. The welts can appear and fade within hours, and the disorder can appear to migrate to different parts of the body.

7. Hives, in addition to itching, can also be painful to the touch and cause a burning or stinging sensation.

8. Hives, when caused by acute urticaria, go away on their own after a few hours to a few days. If the allergen or its trigger still exists, however, symptoms may recur. Hives can stick around for months or even years if you have chronic urticaria.

9. The emotional effects of urticaria include itching that persists despite treatment, the development of hives, and the unpredictable nature of the condition.

Urticaria is a skin ailment that causes itching and redness, and while it can be quite irritating, it is usually not life threatening. In most situations, urticaria can be managed and its symptoms alleviated through treatment, lifestyle changes, and the identification and management of triggers. It's best to see a doctor or dermatologist for an accurate diagnosis and advice on treatment options if you or a loved one are dealing with urticaria.

A healthcare provider, generally a dermatologist or allergist, would conduct a complete evaluation to diagnose urticaria and classify it so that the patient can receive the most effective treatment. **Urticaria is identified and categorized in the following ways:**

1. First, the doctor will ask you a lot of questions about your medical history. They will inquire as to when the symptoms began, how long they lasted, whether there were any triggers or allergies, and if there were any other symptoms, including swelling or breathing difficulties. A complete medical history might assist pinpoint underlying variables and causes.

2. The doctor will do a full body checkup to see how widespread the hives are and how they look on the skin. Angioedema is a similar disorder, so doctors will also be on the lookout for any signs of swelling.

3. Assessment of Allergies: Potential allergens that may be causing the urticaria are identified through a combination of the patient's history and, if necessary, allergy testing (such as skin prick tests or blood tests).

4. Medical professionals treating patients with persistent urticaria may order extra diagnostic procedures to rule out potential causes. This may involve a blood test to detect infections or autoimmune disorders.

5. The diagnosis of physical urticaria (such as cold urticaria or heat urticaria) can be confirmed with the help of physical challenge tests. A cold urticaria test, for instance, uses ice to see if hives form on a small patch of skin.

6. Skin biopsies are occasionally conducted to learn more about the cause of urticarial lesions. This is usually saved for unusual circumstances.

7. Urticaria can be broken down into several categories, such as:

Urticaria is defined as either acute (lasting less than six weeks) or chronic (lasting more than six weeks) depending on its duration.

• **Etiology:** Urticaria is subdivided into types based on the underlying cause or trigger, such as physical (caused by physical stimuli), allergic (triggered by allergens), autoimmune (related to autoimmune responses), and idiopathic (where the cause cannot be identified).

A treatment plan is created after a diagnosis and categorization are made, and it may include changes to one's way of life, the use of antihistamines or other medications, and methods for avoiding triggers. How urticaria is treated depends on the type of urticaria and what is triggering it.

Urticaria: Allergic vs. Non-Allergic

There are two basic forms of urticaria (hives) distinguished by their etiology: allergic urticaria and non-allergic urticaria. The causes of an allergic reaction are used to classify these groups.

1. Allergy Hives:

Allergic urticaria is caused by an immune system reaction to allergens. These allergies can include foods, medications, insect stings, and environmental elements like pollen or dust mites.

Allergic urticaria occurs when the body's immune system reacts to an allergen by releasing histamine and other substances. Hives, or red, itchy welts occur on the skin as a result of this immunological response.

- **Timing:** Allergic urticaria often develops between minutes to hours after contact to the allergen.

Finding and avoiding the allergen that triggers hives is the primary treatment for allergic urticaria. Antihistamines and other drugs may also be used to ease symptoms.

2. Urticaria That Isn't Caused by Allergies

It is important to note that allergic reactions are not the primary driver of non-allergic urticaria, also known as non-immunologic urticaria. It can also be brought on by things that aren't allergens at all, like physical or mental stress, infections, autoimmune factors, or idiopathic (unknown) reasons.

• **Immune Response:** Mast cell activation unrelated to allergies, autoimmune reactions targeting mast cells, and sensitivity to physical variables like pressure, cold, or heat are all potential explanations in non-allergic urticaria.

• **Timing:** The start of non-allergic urticaria can vary based on the exact trigger. When exposed to a physical stimulus, urticaria may manifest very instantly, while urticaria brought on by stress may manifest during or after the stressful event.

In order to effectively treat non-allergic urticaria, it is necessary to first pinpoint what is causing it. Antihistamines, changes in lifestyle, and other drugs may all be used to treat and manage chronic urticaria.

The treatment and management of allergic and non-allergic urticaria are very different, therefore it's crucial to get the diagnosis right the first time. A healthcare physician, allergist, or dermatologist should be consulted for a definitive diagnosis and individualized treatment strategy in both circumstances.

CHAPTER THREE
Overcoming Severe Urticaria

Hives that persist fewer than six weeks are considered acute urticaria, and their management entails symptom management, avoiding triggers, and getting medical attention if necessary. In order to deal with acute urticaria, try the following:

1. Recognize and Sidestep Triggers:

• Consider whether any recent changes in your lifestyle, nutrition, or exposures could be to blame for the rash.

• Maintain a journal detailing your exposure to new goods, substances, and foods, as well as the times and days that you get hives. Possible causes can be determined with this method.

2. Consume Antihistamines:

• Itching and the severity of hives can be alleviated by over-the-counter antihistamines (such as loratadine, cetirizine, or fexofenadine. To ensure proper dose, refer to the product label or consult your healthcare provider.

3. Skin injury or infection may result from scratching, which can also make urticaria worse. Don't scratch the irritated areas if you can help it.

4. A Cold Compress Can Help:

• Hives can be soothed with the application of cool, wet compresses, which also have the added benefit of reducing inflammation.

5. Put on Loose Clothes:

• Wearing clothes that fit loosely and allow air to circulate will help prevent skin irritation.

6. Avoiding Common Allergens:

• If you have hives and you think a certain allergen (food, medication, etc.) is to blame, you should avoid that allergen until you can see a doctor.

7. Avoid dehydration:

• Hydration is an important factor in skin maintenance. To maintain healthy skin, a regular water intake is essential.

8. Stress can increase hives. Try deep breathing, meditation, or yoga to calm your mind and body and reduce your tension.

9. Get in Touch with Your Doctor:

• Seek professional help if your hives are severe, persistent, or do not improve after using over-the-counter antihistamines. A doctor will be able to determine what's causing your acute urticaria, what medication will work best, and how to administer it.

10. Extreme hives can signal a potentially fatal allergic reaction known as anaphylaxis. Seek emergency medical assistance if you have trouble breathing, facial or throat swelling, disorientation, or a drop in blood pressure.

Keep in mind that acute urticaria usually goes away if the triggering factor is eliminated or treated. Chronic urticaria is diagnosed when hives last longer than six weeks or return regularly, indicating the need for additional investigation.

If your hives are severe or persistent, you should see a doctor to get advice and to rule out more serious problems.

Alternative Treatments

Urticaria (hives) can be treated in a number of ways, depending on the severity, nature, and origin of the problem. Urticaria can be efficiently treated and controlled by a number of methods. Some of the most often used treatments are as follows:

1. Antihistamines:

The most common treatment for urticaria is antihistamines. Hives are brought on by a substance called histamine, which is generated in the body after an allergic reaction and is what these pills aim to counteract. Many patients get relief from these symptoms after using an OTC antihistamine such loratadine, cetirizine, or fexofenadine. Prescription antihistamines may be required in some instances.

2. Antihistamines may be used in conjunction with H2 blockers such ranitidine and cimetidine to reduce symptoms. Their mechanism for preventing histamine's effects is unique.

3. Corticosteroids:

Short-term usage of oral corticosteroids (such as prednisone) may be administered in severe cases or when antihistamines alone are ineffective. Long-term usage of corticosteroids is not suggested owing to potential side effects, however short-term use can help reduce inflammation and alleviate symptoms fast.

4. Anaphylaxis medication epinephrine:

Epinephrine is used as a life-saving emergency treatment in cases of severe allergic reactions or anaphylaxis. This calls for rapid medical attention and is typically treated with an auto-injector (EpiPen).

5. Auto injector:

Some people with chronic urticaria may be given an epinephrine auto-injector to carry with them at all times in case of a severe allergic reaction or anaphylaxis.

6. Immunosuppressant:

Some people with chronic urticaria may benefit from immunosuppressive drugs like cyclosporine or mycophenolate mofetil if other treatments have failed. In some people with chronic urticaria, these medications help reduce the autoimmune reaction.

7. Biologics:

• The biologic medicine omalizumab (Xolair) has been licensed for the treatment of patients with chronic idiopathic urticaria who have not found relief from previous therapies. It prevents allergies by attacking the IgE antibody.

8. Adjustments to Your Way of Life:

It's crucial to zero in on causes and steer clear of them. This could involve alterations to one's eating habits, personal care routine, or surrounding environment. Preventative interventions against physical triggers can help with physical urticaria.

9. Other Treatment Options:

Herbal medicines and acupuncture are two alternative treatments that some urticaria sufferers try, although the evidence for their efficacy is mixed. Before taking any alternative remedies, talk to your doctor.

10. Help for the Mind:

Living with chronic urticaria can be stressful mentally. Stress and anxiety caused by the disease can be managed with the help of counseling or other forms of psychological support.

The best course of treatment for your urticaria and its underlying causes can be determined by speaking with a healthcare professional, generally a dermatologist or allergist. Your reaction to treatment and the dynamic nature of your condition may necessitate a combination of treatment modalities.

CHAPTER FOUR
Reasons Why and How to Avoid It

One of the most important parts of urticaria management is learning to recognize and avoid your condition's triggers. It's vital to pay attention to one's personal experiences and engage with a healthcare physician to identify particular causes, as triggers might vary from person to person.

1. Allergens:

• Foods, drugs, insect stings, and environmental variables like pollen, dust mites, and pet dander can all behave as allergens due to their potential to set off an allergic reaction. Prevention:

Gets allergy testing from a specialist if you think a specific allergen is to blame for your hives.

Once allergies have been identified, avoidance is the best way of protection. Altering one's diet, switching to allergy-free alternatives, or taking other measures to lessen ambient allergen exposure could all be part of the solution.

2. External Variables:

Physical urticaria can be produced by pressure, cold, heat, friction, or vibrations, among other physical stimuli. Prevention:

• Wearing warm clothing, utilizing heated blankets, and avoiding extreme temperature fluctuations will alleviate cold urticaria symptoms.

• If you suffer from heat urticaria, it may help to use air conditioning.

Wear loose clothing and try not to stay in one position for too long if you suffer from pressure urticaria.

• Avoidance of certain physical stimuli is the key preventative technique.

3. Stress:

Urticaria can be made worse by emotional stress in some people. Prevention:

• Relaxation exercises, mindfulness, meditation, or therapy are all great stress management approaches that can help lessen the negative effects of stress on urticaria.

Prevention relies on awareness and management of personal stressors.

4. Medications:

Urticaria can be triggered by taking certain pharmaceuticals such antibiotics or nonsteroidal anti-inflammatory drugs (NSAIDs). Prevention:

Inform your doctor if you've ever developed hives after using a certain drug. They may suggest other drugs to try.

• Tell your doctor if you have any allergies or sensitivities to medications.

5. Infections:

Infections are a possible cause of urticaria. Prevention:

Good cleanliness and vaccines can lessen the likelihood of contracting infectious diseases.

Reducing the likelihood of urticaria is also possible by prompt treatment and management of infections.

6. Autoimmune Origins:

Causes The immune system may attack the body's own mast cells in cases of autoimmune urticaria. Prevention:

• Identifying and controlling autoimmune causes through medication and therapy under the advice of a healthcare specialist is vital.

7. Isolated Incidents:

Causes Urticaria can have unknown or unidentified causes (idiopathic). Prevention:

• Medication and lifestyle changes are aimed for symptom management and preventing repeated outbreaks in idiopathic instances.

Consult a doctor, such as an allergist or dermatologist, to figure out what sets off your symptoms and create a treatment plan tailored to you. The key to preventing repeated hives and properly managing the condition is making some changes to one's lifestyle, avoiding recognized triggers, and sticking to the suggested treatment plan.

Urticaria: Daily Life

The unpredictability and discomfort of urticaria make it difficult to live with either type of the ailment. People with urticaria face unique challenges, but with the correct methods and support, they can live happy and productive lives. If you suffer with urticaria, consider the following advice:

• If you haven't seen a dermatologist or an allergist yet,

you should. They can give you an accurate diagnosis and recommend a suitable course of therapy. Working with a healthcare provider is vital for controlling urticaria properly.

• If your doctor has prescribed a certain course of treatment, be sure to stick to it. Depending on the severity of your symptoms, your doctor may recommend antihistamines, prescription drugs, or other treatments.

• Pay close attention to your body and environment in order to discover triggers that lead to hives, and take steps to avoid them. Once these causes have been recognized, preventative measures can be taken to stop epidemics.

• Keeping a symptom diary might help you identify triggers for your hives, including certain foods, medications, and times of day they occur. Your doctor may find this information helpful.

• Hives can be caused by stress, so it's important to learn stress-management practices like meditation, yoga, and breathing exercises.

• Overall skin health can be supported by drinking plenty of water and eating a healthy, well-balanced diet.

• Dress for comfort by donning loose-fitting garments crafted from natural, breathable fabrics that won't chafe or restrict movement.

• Wet, cool compresses can be applied to hives to reduce inflammation and irritation.

•.Don't Scratch! Scratching hives can make the rash worse and can cause infection if you break the skin.

• Emotional support: coping with chronic urticaria can be difficult. If you need help, talk to somebody you trust or join a group. The emotional toll of this ailment can be lessened with counseling or therapy.

• Learn as much as you can about urticaria, what causes it, and what medications can help you manage your symptoms. You will be better able to deal with your condition if you increase your level of knowledge about it.

• When traveling, bring any necessary drugs with you, such as antihistamines or an epinephrine auto-injector, if you suffer from chronic urticaria or are at risk for severe allergic responses.

- In the event of a severe allergic response, it is imperative that you and your loved ones are familiar with the usage of an epinephrine auto-injector.

- Follow-Up sessions It is important to schedule follow-up sessions with your doctor to check in on your progress and make any required adjustments to your treatment plan.

- **Be Patient:** Urticaria might be annoying, but it often improves over time. Allow your treatment to take effect gradually.

It's important to remember that most people with urticaria can find relief from their symptoms with the right treatment and management, and that they can continue to enjoy a high quality of life despite living with this condition. Don't be shy about seeking assistance from doctors and other people in your community if you're struggling to control your urticaria symptoms.

Concerns Unique to Urticaria in Children

Hives, or urticaria, can afflict both children and adults. It is important to take the child's comfort and safety into account when treating pediatric urticaria. When dealing with pediatric urticaria, it is crucial to bear in mind the following:

1. If your child has urticaria, you should see a pediatrician or a pediatric dermatologist who specializes in treating children. Children should see a pediatrician or pediatric dermatologist for diagnosis and treatment.

2. Medication Dosing for Children Doctors often prescribe antihistamines dosable by a child's age and weight when treating urticaria in children. Take drugs exactly as prescribed and discuss any drug interactions or adverse effects with your child's pediatrician.

3. Liquid or chewable tablet versions should be offered for medications to make dosing and administration simpler for children.

4. Urticaria in children can be prevented by learning to recognize and avoid the triggers that bring on an attack. Keep a vigilant eye on potential allergies in their environment, especially foods and common allergens like insect stings.

5. Stress, like in adults, can make urticaria worse in kids. Here's how to deal with it. Play, relaxation exercises, and imaginative play are all great stress management approaches that are appropriate for children.

6. Educate the youngster: Talk to the youngster about their illness in terms he or she can grasp. Inspire them to keep an eye out for and report any signs of distress.

7. Avoid Skin Damage and Infection by Discouraging Scratching Have parents discourage their children from scratching their hives. It could assist if their nails were trimmed and they slept with soft mittens.

8. Children should be dressed in loose, breathable clothing to help prevent chafing. Pick soft fabrics like cotton that won't irritate your skin.

9. Kids' skin health can benefit from a variety of lifestyle choices, including those related to hydration and nutrition.

10. Keep an eye out for anaphylaxis, and make sure the child's parents, caregivers, and teachers know how to use an epinephrine auto-injector if he or she is at risk for severe allergic reactions or anaphylaxis.

11. Join a community that specializes in helping kids who suffer with urticaria and other allergic reactions. Both children and their parents can benefit from the knowledge and comfort that these materials bring.

12. Follow-up appointments with the pediatrician should be scheduled on a regular basis so that the child's progress can be monitored and the treatment plan adjusted as needed.

Both children and their parents may experience distress when dealing with pediatric urticaria. Helping children with urticaria maintain healthy and happy lives requires open communication with the healthcare practitioner, the creation of a supportive atmosphere at home and school, and the use of age-appropriate techniques to educating and managing the illness.

Conclusion

Hives, or urticaria, is an acute skin reaction that causes red, itchy bumps to form suddenly. Allergens, physical triggers, stress, infections, and autoimmune responses are just some of the things that might bring on this condition. Different approaches are needed for diagnosing and treating acute and chronic urticaria.

• Antihistamines, corticosteroids, and other, more specialist drugs are commonly used for treatment after a comprehensive evaluation by a healthcare provider has established a diagnosis. Modifications to one's way of life, including the recognition and avoidance of urticaria triggers, the control of stress, and the practice of good hygiene, are essential for the management of this condition.

• With the help of a doctor, the encouragement of loved ones, and regular application of medication, people with urticaria can lead productive lives with minimal interference from their hives.

Age-appropriate therapy, communication, and child-friendly stress management approaches are particularly important for pediatric urticaria.

In order to properly treat urticaria and guarantee the best possible quality of life for yourself or your kid, it is crucial to seek medical advice, collaborate with healthcare specialists, and keep educated.

THE END